8 DIMENSIONS

of

HEALTH AND

WELLNESS

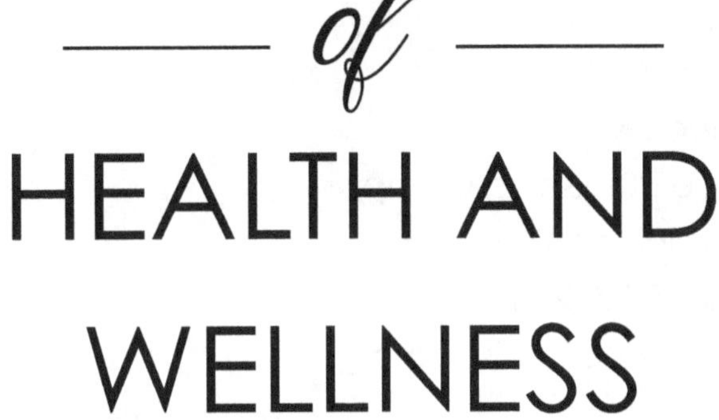

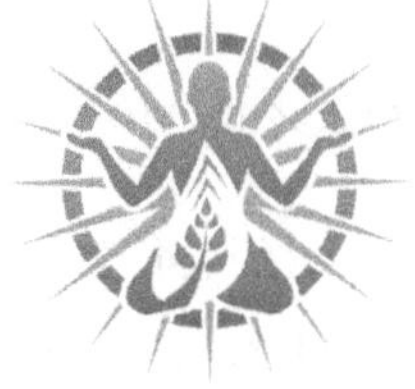

Coach Te

www.TrueVinePublishing.org

8 Dimensions of Health and Wellness
Coach Te

Published by
True Vine Publishing Company
810 Dominican Dr.
Nashville TN 37228
www.TrueVinePublishing.org

ISBN: 978-1-968092-49-8 Paperback
ISBN: 978-1-968092-50-4 eBook

Printed in the United States of America–First Print

For more info go to www.MyTreeofTranquility.com

TABLE OF CONTENTS

Welcome to Your Journey of Wholeness

Health is more than just the absence of illness; it is a vibrant state of being that involves every part of who you are. Often, we focus so much on our physical bodies that we overlook the other pillars that keep us upright.

This booklet is designed around the 8 Dimensions of Wellness: Physical, Emotional, Social, Spiritual, Intellectual, Occupational, Environmental, and Financial. True "well-being" happens when we find a sustainable harmony between all of them.

Why This Book was Written

We live in a fast-paced world where it is easy to feel "off-balance" without knowing why. You might be physically fit but feel socially isolated, or financially secure but emotionally drained. This book was created to help you identify those gaps. The goal is to get each of us to move away from "quick fixes" and toward a lifestyle of intention. By exploring these eight dimensions, you can discover which areas of your life need more nourishment and which areas of your life are already thriving.

How to use this booklet

This booklet is not a textbook to be read once and put away to collect dust. This is a workbook for your life. Here is how to get the most out of it:

1. Start with a Self-assessment. Check in with yourself and be honest.

2. Focus on one Dimension at a time. Don't feel pressured to overhaul all eight areas at once. Choose the one that feels most urgent or interesting to you and start there.

3. Use the "Action Steps" Set small achievable goals. Write in your personal notes in the space provided.

4. Revisit Regularly. Wellness is a practice, not a destination. Come back to these pages every few months to see how your balance has shifted.

Remember, small consistent changes lead to the most significant transformations. We invite you to turn the page with an open mind and a commitment to your most vibrant self.

EMOTIONAL WELLNESS

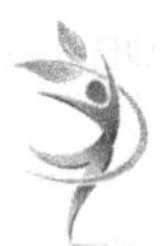

Emotional wellness is the ability to acknowledge, understand, and process emotions in a healthy way. It requires honesty with yourself first. Many of us were taught to suppress our feelings, minimize our pain, or stay strong for others, often at the expense of our own well-being. Emotional wellness invites you to stop running from your emotions and instead sit with them gently.

This dimension teaches that emotions are not problems to fix but messages to understand. Anger, sadness, fear, and joy all have value. When we allow ourselves to feel without judgment, we create space for healing.

Emotional wellness means taking the time for Emotional checks and recognizing when support is needed. An Emotional check is a deliberate practice of pausing to identify, acknowledge, and name your current feelings. There is no judgment involved.

Emotional checks help to facilitate healthy coping strategies. Healthy coping strategies are intentional actions used to manage stress, painful emotions, and difficult situations.

Unlike "numbing" behaviors like excessive scrolling or overeating, healthy strategies help you process the emotion so it can eventually dissipate.

An Emotional check in is a deliberate practice of pausing to identify, acknowledge, and name your current feelings. There is no judgment involved.

Some examples of Healthy coping strategies are:

1. Physical Coping - The Bottom Up approach

2. Cognitive Coping - The Top Down approach

3. Social & Spiritual Coping

4. Creative & Intellectual Coping

With emotional wellness, resilience replaces reactivity. You become better equipped to navigate stress, set boundaries, and respond thoughtfully instead of reacting impulsively. Emotional balance creates inner safety, and inner safety creates peace.

🪷 Reflection Questions 🪷

What emotions do I avoid?

____

____

____

____

How do I manage stress?

____

____

____

____

🌼 Action Steps 🌼

Practice emotional check-ins.

Use one healthy coping strategy.

PHYSICAL WELLNESS

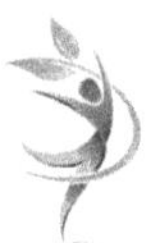

Physical wellness is often where we first notice imbalance, yet it is the dimension we most commonly push aside. Our bodies quietly carry our stress, exhaustion, and unprocessed emotions long before we are willing to acknowledge them. When we ignore our physical needs, the body finds ways to speak: through fatigue, pain, illness, or burnout. Physical wellness is not about perfection or appearance; it is about learning to listen with compassion and respond with care.

Honoring your body means recognizing that rest is not weakness, movement is not punishment, and nourishment is not something to earn. Each choice to hydrate, stretch, sleep, or slow down is an act of self-respect. Physical wellness asks us to rebuild trust with our bodies, especially if that trust has been broken through overwork, stress, or neglect.

When the body feels supported, life feels more manageable. Energy increases, clarity improves, and resilience strengthens. Physical wellness becomes the foundation that allows all other dimensions of wellness to grow.

Physical Wellness supports the body through movement, rest, nourishment, and preventive care.

🪷 Reflection Questions 🪷

How do I care for my body daily?

____

____

____

____

What physical habits need improvement?

____

____

____

____

🌿 Action Steps 🌿

Move intentionally 3x weekly.

Improve hydration or sleep.

INTELLECTUAL WELLNESS

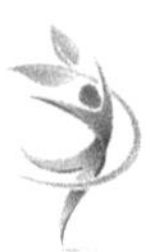

Intellectual wellness is about curiosity, openness, and the willingness to learn about the world and about yourself. It invites you to challenge old beliefs, expand your understanding, and remain mentally engaged throughout life. Growth happens when we allow ourselves to question what we have been taught and make room for new perspectives.

Many people confuse intellectual wellness with academic achievement, but it is much deeper than that. It is the courage to think critically, reflect honestly, and remain mentally flexible. Intellectual wellness thrives when we give ourselves permission to evolve, change our minds, and grow beyond outdated narratives.

When intellectual wellness is nurtured, confidence grows. You begin to trust your judgment, explore ideas without fear, and engage in meaningful conversations. Learning becomes empowering rather than intimidating, and curiosity becomes a tool for healing and expansion. Intellectual Wellness Promotes learning, curiosity, and mental growth.

🪷 Reflection Questions 🪷

How do you stimulate your mind?

____

____

____

____

How do you open your mind to new ideas?

____

____

____

____

🌿 Action Steps 🌿

Read weekly.

Journal reflections.

SOCIAL WELLNESS

Social wellness is rooted in connection, belonging, and the quality of our relationships. Humans are not meant to exist in isolation, yet many people feel deeply alone even when surrounded by others. Social wellness asks us to evaluate not just who is around us, but how those relationships make us feel.

Healthy relationships offer support, respect, and authenticity. They allow you to be seen without shrinking yourself or performing for acceptance. Social wellness also involves learning to communicate honestly, establish boundaries, and let go of relationships that no longer serve your growth.

When social wellness is strong, you feel supported rather than drained. You learn that connection does not require self-sacrifice and that meaningful relationships are built on mutual care and understanding.

Social Wellness strengthens connection, communication, and belonging.

Which relationships energize me?

____

____

____

____

How do I honor my boundaries and the boundaries of others?

____

____

____

____

🌿 Action Steps 🌿

Nurture one relationship.

Practice setting boundaries for the day.

SPIRITUAL WELLNESS

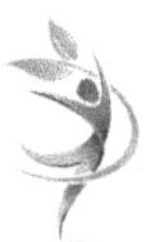

Spiritual wellness is about connection to something greater than yourself, to your values, or to a sense of purpose and meaning. It is deeply personal and unique to each individual. For some, it is rooted in faith; for others, it is found in nature, reflection, or service. Spiritual wellness offers grounding in times of uncertainty.

This dimension provides a sense of inner alignment. It helps you understand who you are beyond titles, roles, and responsibilities. Spiritual wellness encourages stillness, reflection, and intentional living, especially in a world that constantly demands movement and productivity.

When spiritual wellness is nurtured, life feels more purposeful. You gain clarity in decision-making, peace in uncertainty, and strength during challenges. It becomes an anchor that keeps you grounded, no matter what season you are in. Spiritual Wellness fosters purpose, meaning, and grounding.

✿ Reflection Questions ✿

What gives my life meaning?

____

____

____

____

How do I stay grounded?

____

____

____

____

✿ Action Steps ✿

Practice gratitude.

Reflect on values.

ENVIRONMENTAL WELLNESS

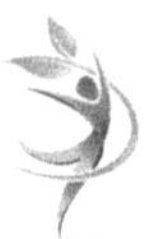

Environmental wellness focuses on the spaces you live, work, and exist in and how they influence your mental and emotional state. Cluttered, chaotic, or unsafe environments can quietly increase stress and anxiety. Our surroundings matter more than we often realize.

This dimension invites you to intentionally create spaces that promote calm, focus, and comfort. Environmental wellness is not about perfection; it is about awareness. It asks what your environment communicates to your nervous system and how it supports—or disrupts—your peace.

When your environment feels safe and supportive, your mind can rest. A peaceful space becomes a reflection of inner balance and provides room for clarity, creativity, and healing.

Environmental wellness creates supportive, calming environments.

🪷 Reflection Questions 🪷

How does my space promote peace?

____

____

____

____

What needs decluttering in my environment?

____

____

____

____

🌼 Action Steps 🌼

Organize one area.

Add calming elements.

OCCUPATIONAL WELLNESS

Occupational wellness reflects your relationship with work, purpose, and fulfillment. It is not only about employment but about whether your daily efforts align with your values and well-being. Many people stay in survival mode at work, sacrificing health and peace for stability, often without realizing the toll it takes.

This dimension encourages balance between ambition and rest, contribution and self-care. Occupational wellness asks whether your work energizes you or depletes you, and whether boundaries exist to protect your time, health, and identity.

When occupational wellness is aligned, work becomes meaningful rather than draining. You feel valued, respected, and supported, and your sense of purpose extends beyond productivity alone.

Occupational Wellness Aligns purpose, fulfillment, and work-life balance.

🪷 Reflection Questions 🪷

Do I feel aligned at work? If not, why?

____

____

____

____

What causes burnout for me?

____

____

____

____

🌿 Action Steps 🌿

Create a list of boundaries that will help you avoid frustration and burnout.

Seek coaching support.

FINANCIAL WELLNESS

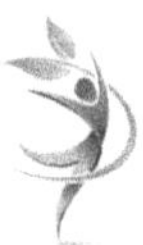

Financial wellness is not solely about how much money you have; it is about your relationship with money. It includes awareness, confidence, planning, and emotional safety. Financial stress can quietly impact mental, emotional, and physical health, often creating cycles of anxiety and avoidance.

This dimension encourages honesty and empowerment. Financial wellness grows when we replace fear with understanding and avoidance with intention. It is about learning to manage finances in a way that supports stability, freedom, and peace.

When financial wellness is nurtured, stress decreases and confidence increases. You gain clarity, make informed decisions, and create a future that feels secure rather than overwhelming.

Financial wellness builds clarity, confidence, and stability around finances.

🪷 Reflection Questions 🪷

How do finances affect my stress level?

____

____

____

____

How have I been proactive or avoidant concerning my financial wellness?

____

____

____

____

🪷 Action Steps 🪷

Review finances.

Set one financial goal.

Notes

Notes

Notes

Notes

Notes

Notes

Notes

Notes

Notes

Notes

Notes

Notes

Notes